This Journal Belongs To:

_____

choose JOY

Life wants what is best for me. I am ok right now

_____

_____

_____

_____

_____

_____

_____

_____

_____

_____

_____

_____

_____

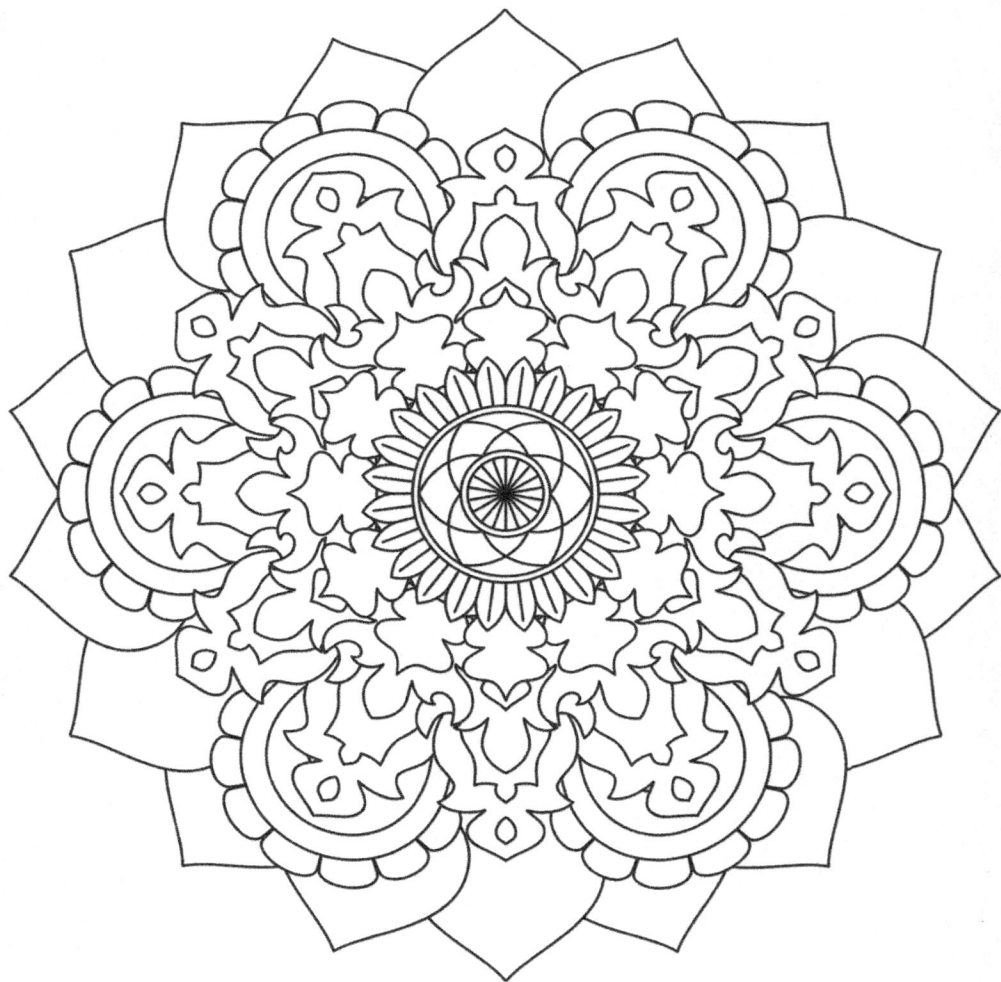

I can find pleasure in my life right now

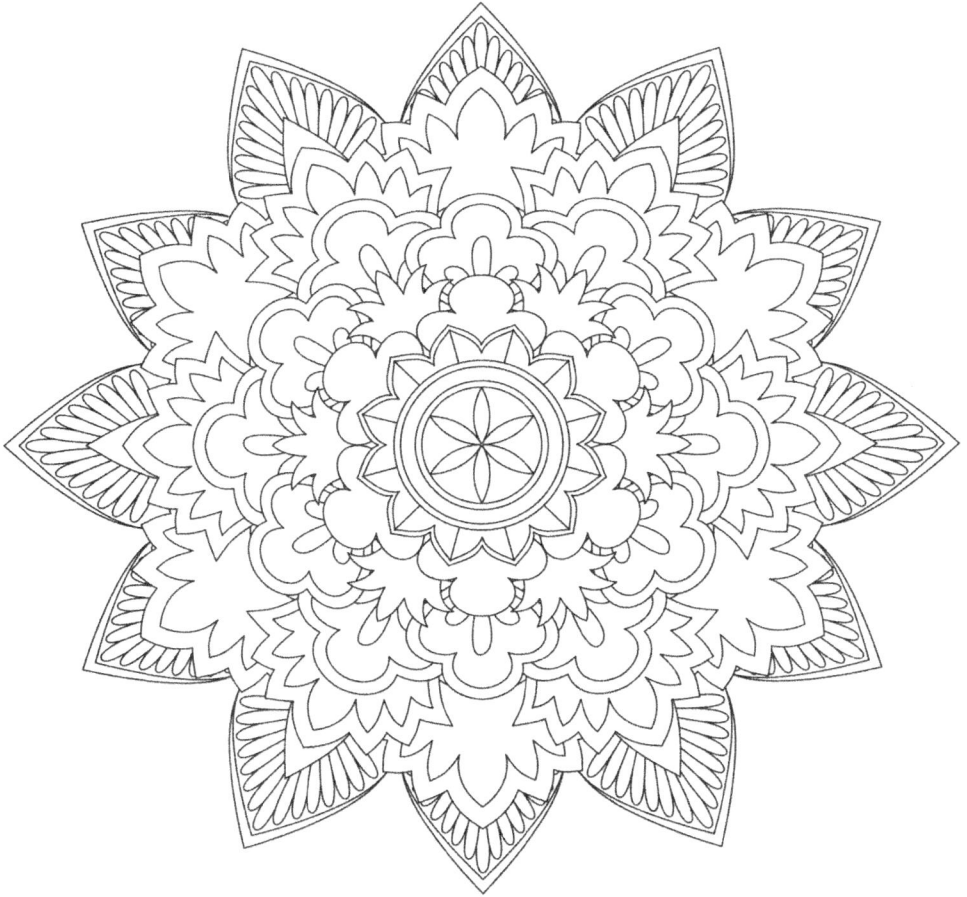

I am relaxed. I am calm

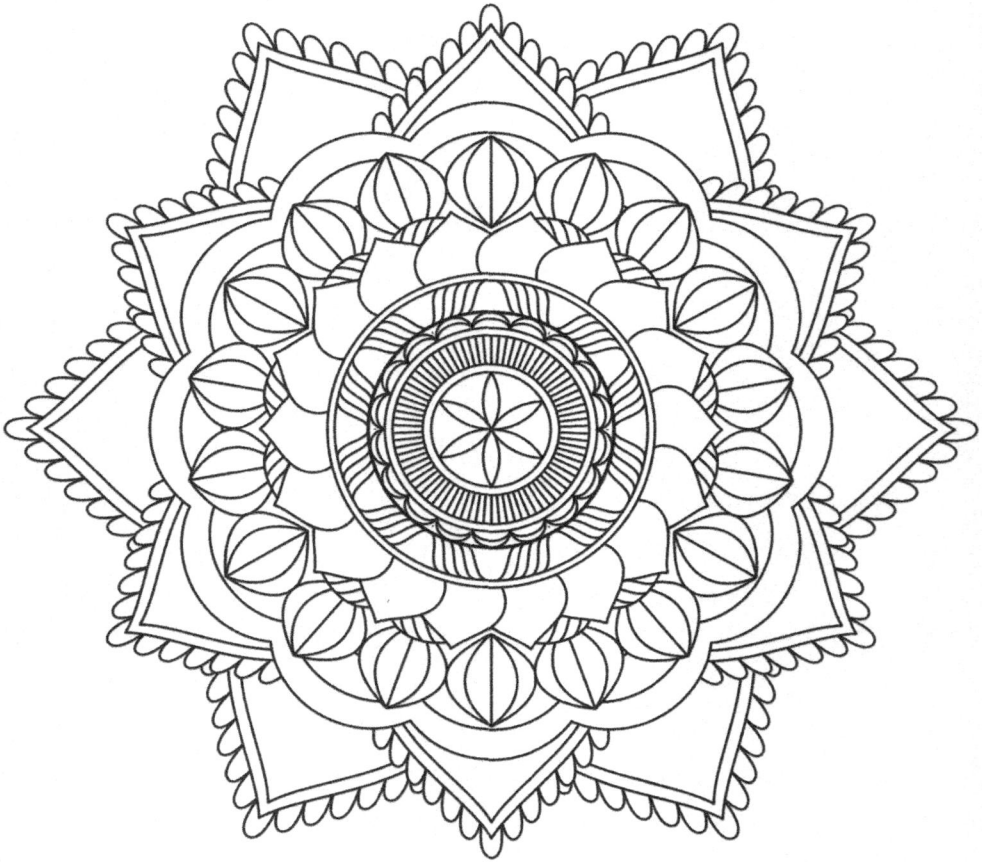

I am free from anxiety. I am in control

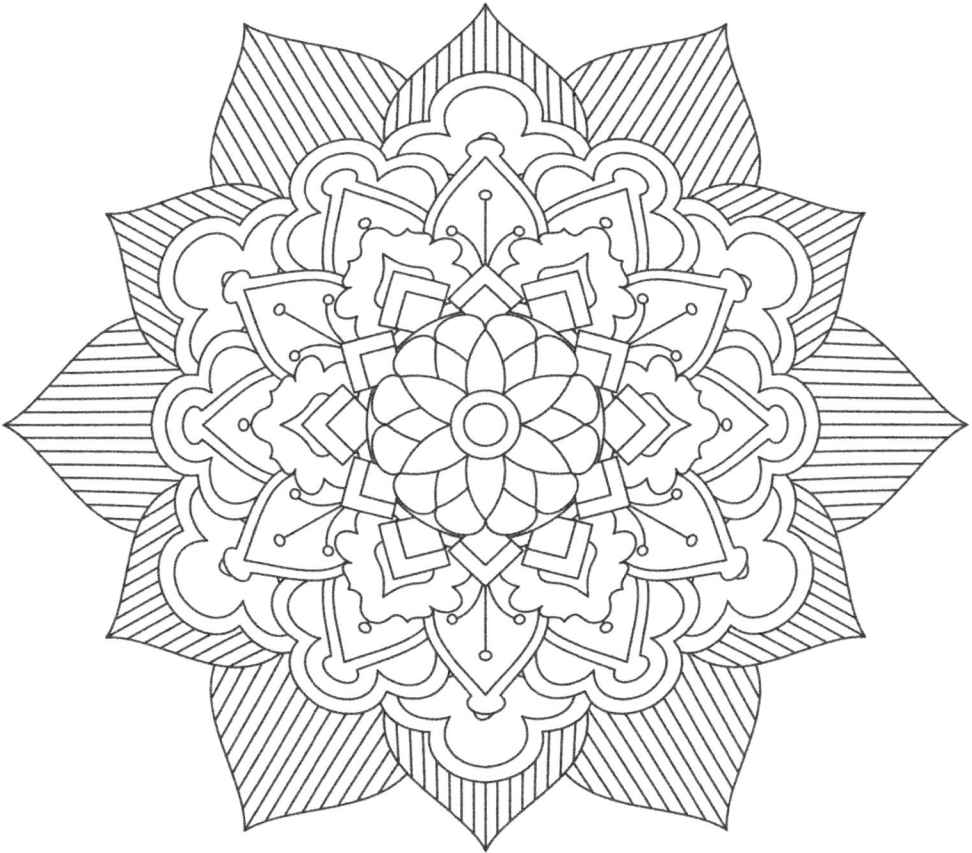

I can do this.

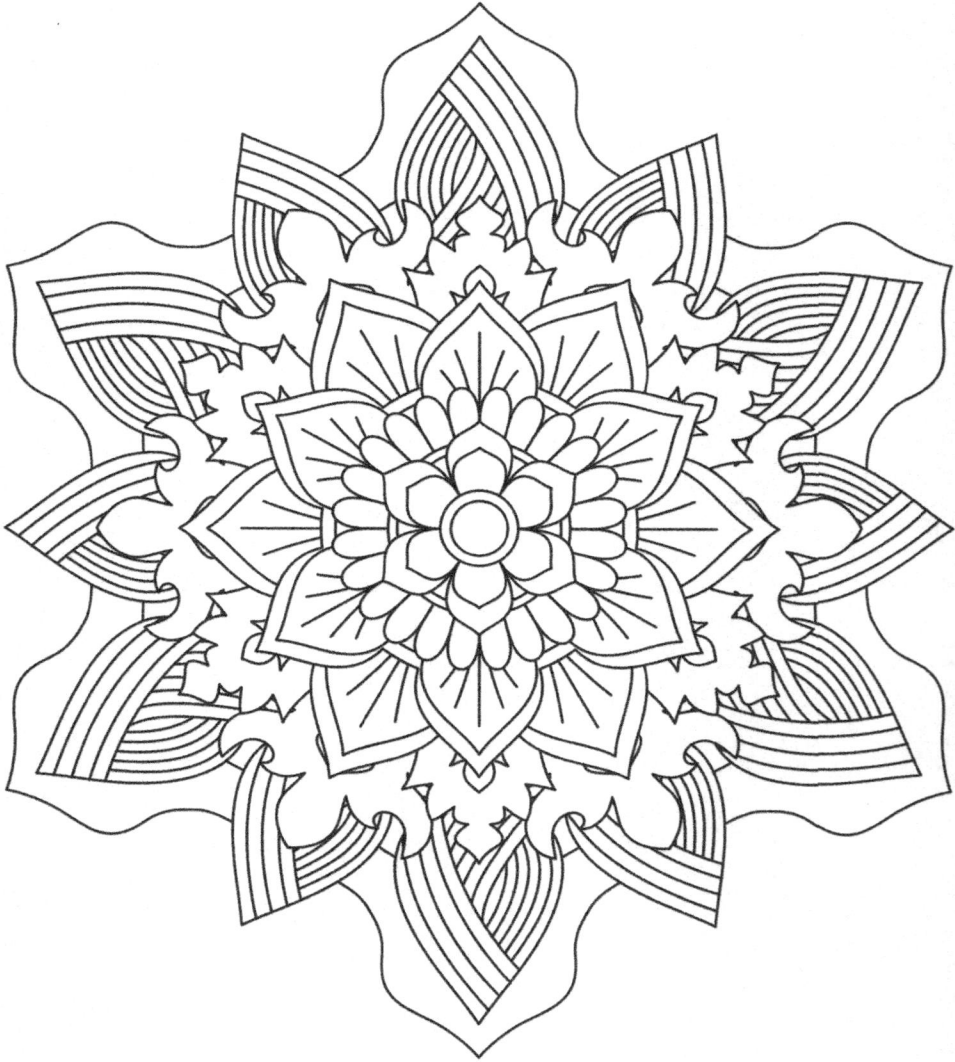

It's okay to take things one step at a time

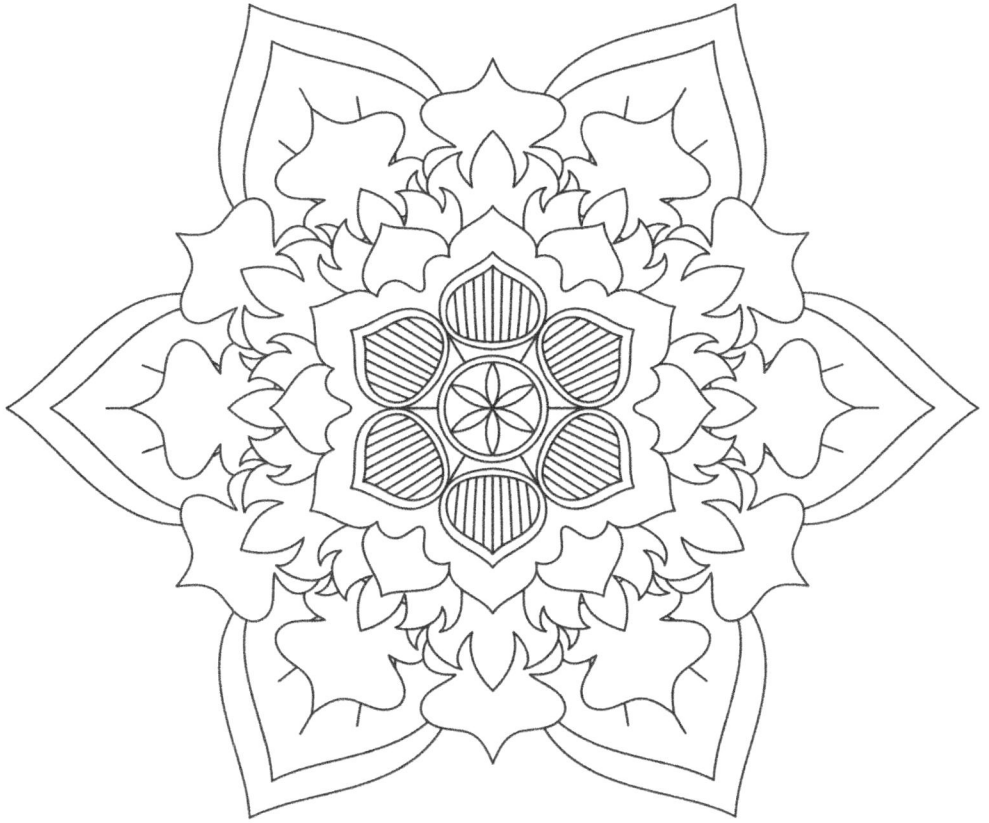

I'm courageous and can make it through

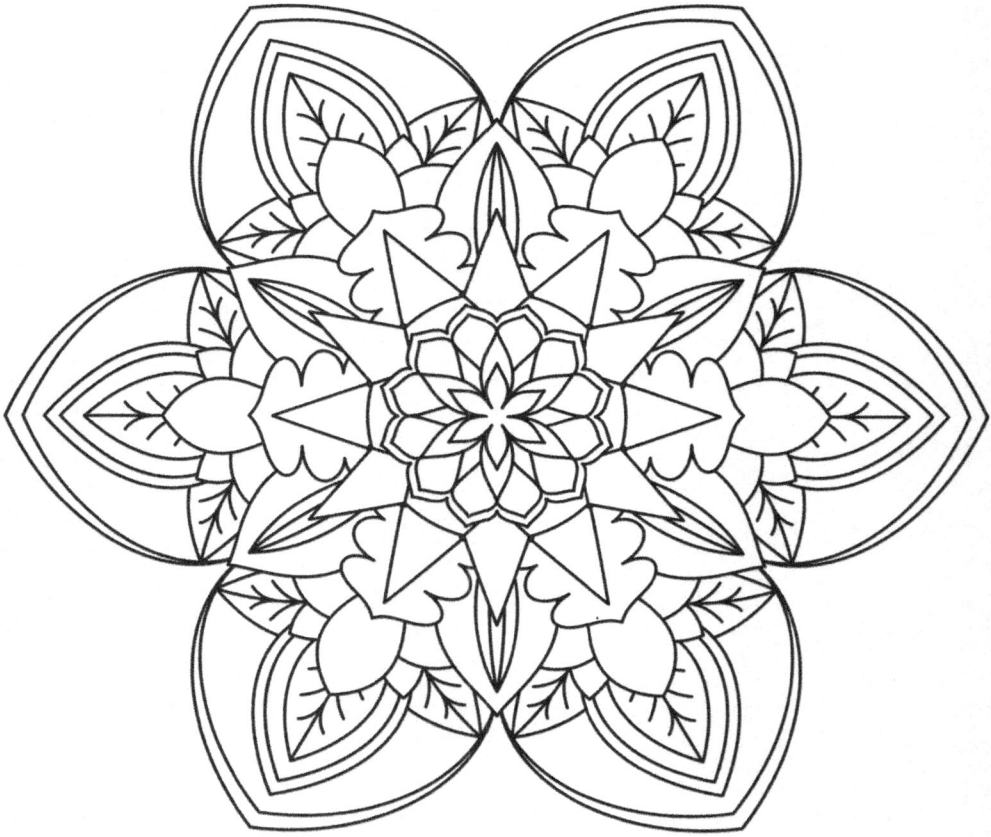

I live only in this moment

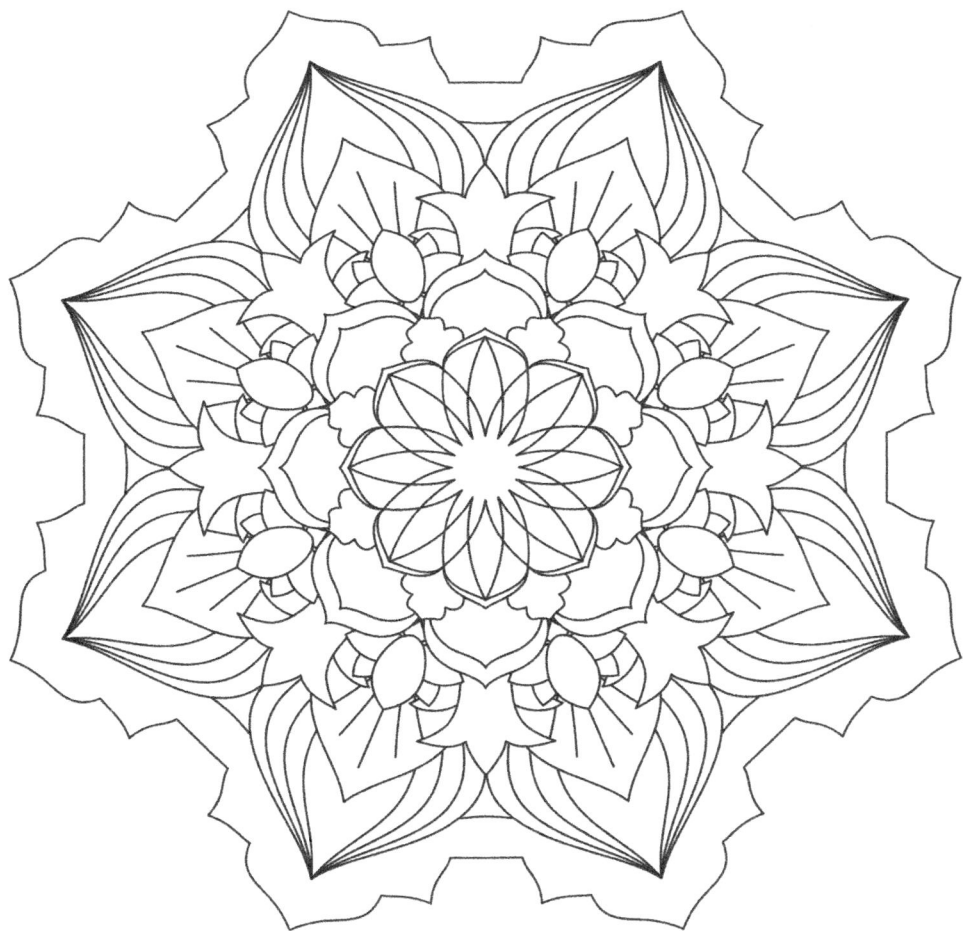

I know everything will work out

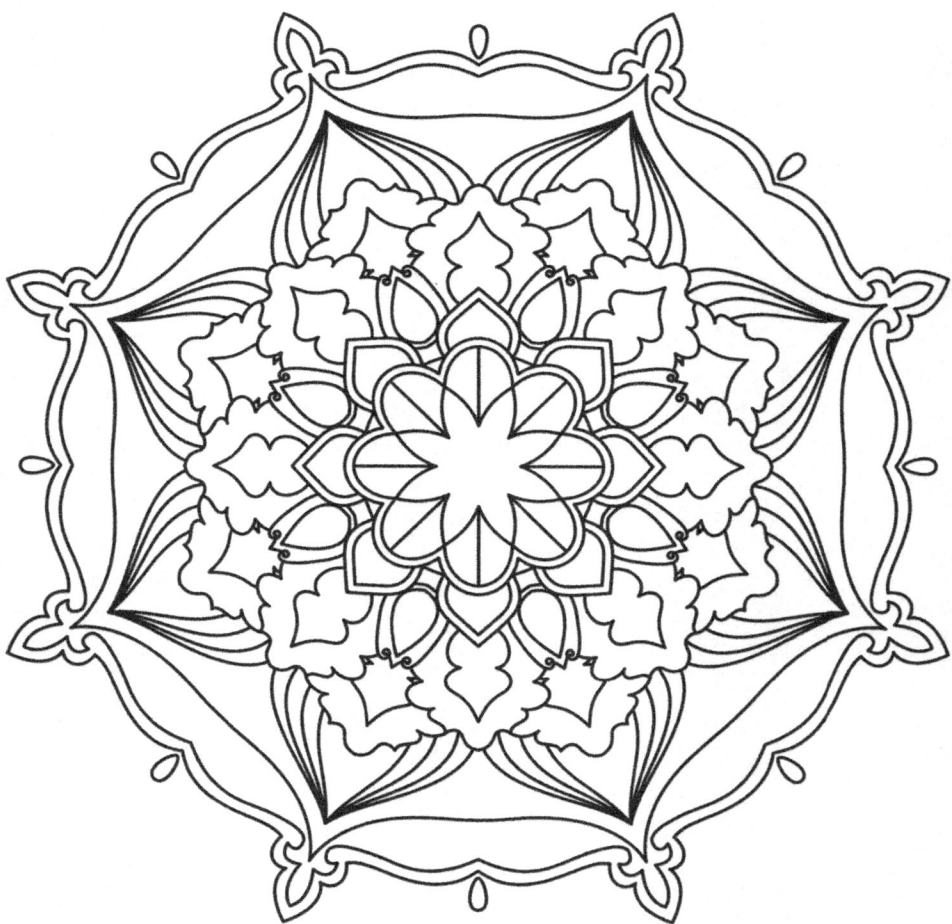

I am not alone in my struggles

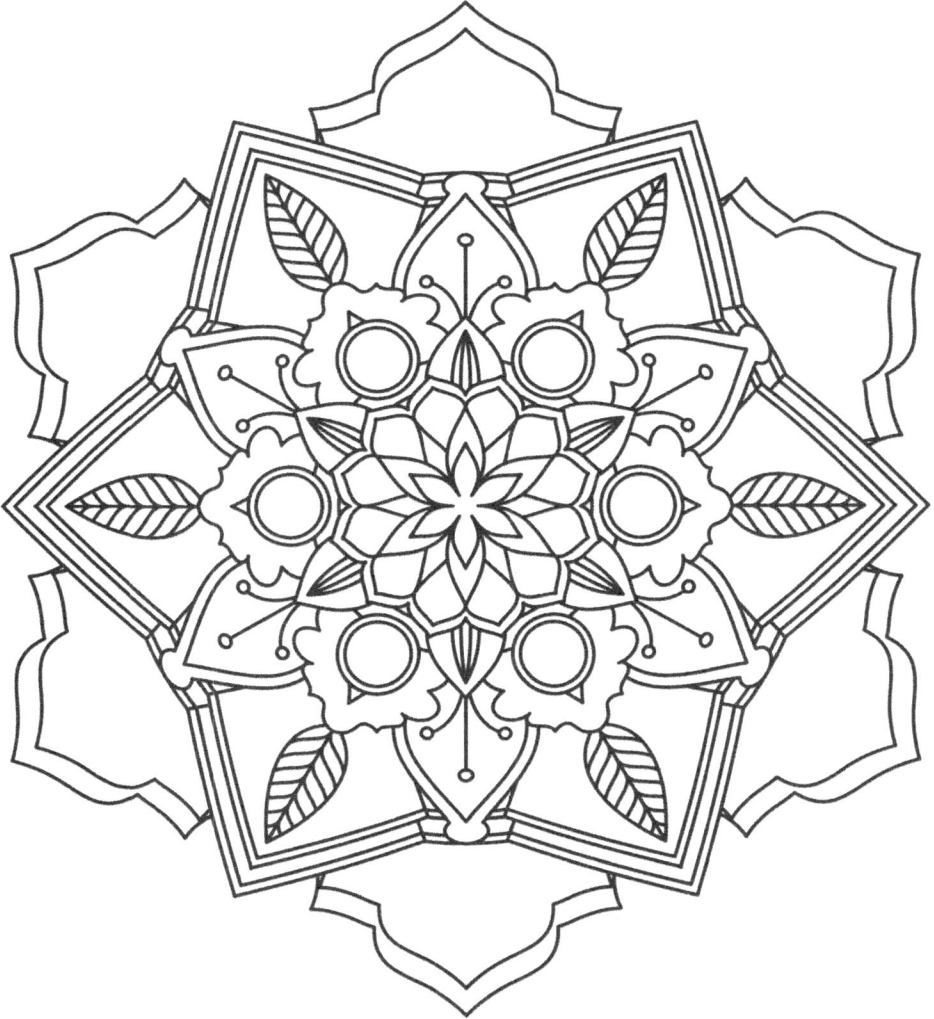

Every breath I take fills my soul with ease

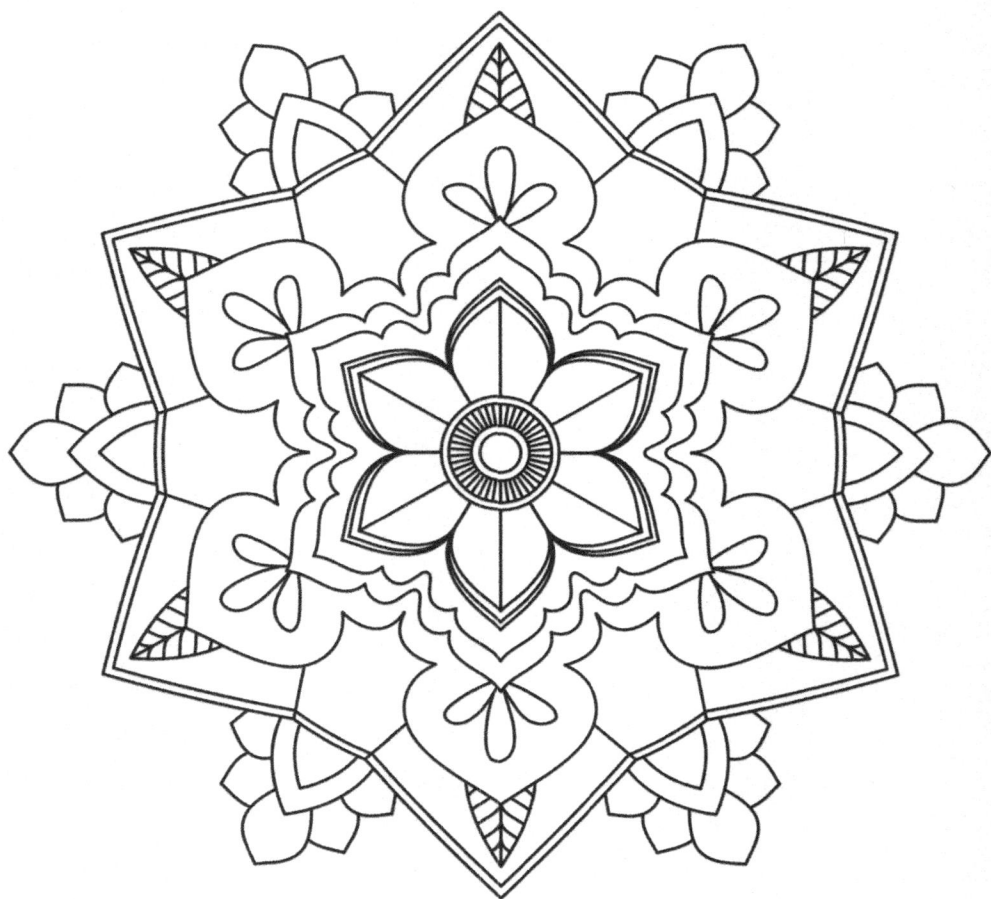

I can climb the biggest mountain

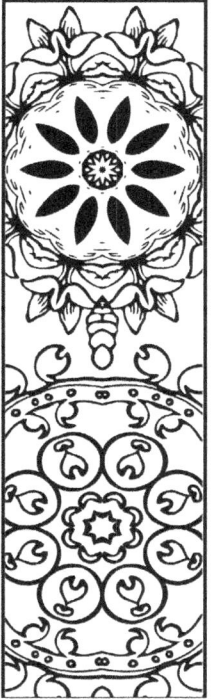

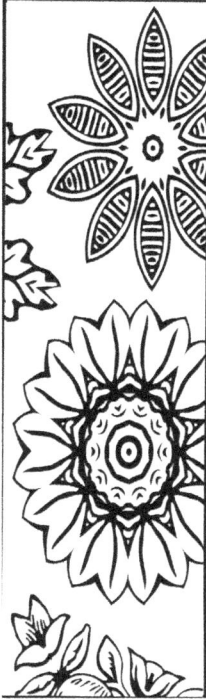

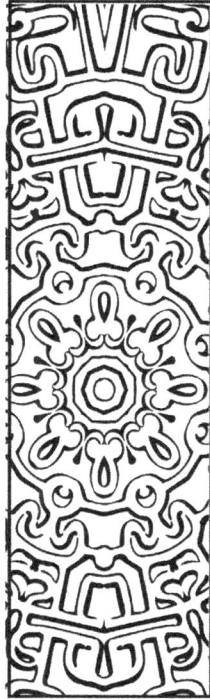

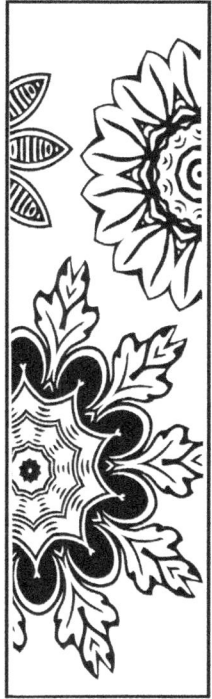

I don't have to be perfect. I just have to be me

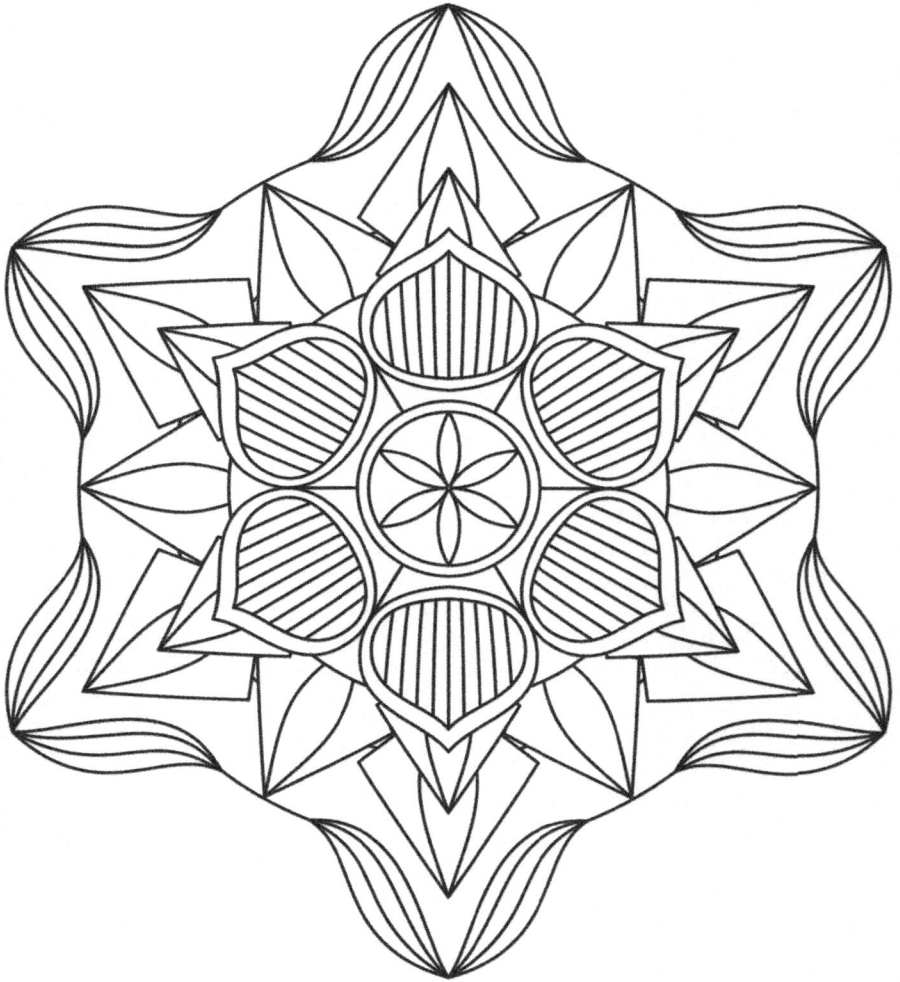

I have the power to live my dreams

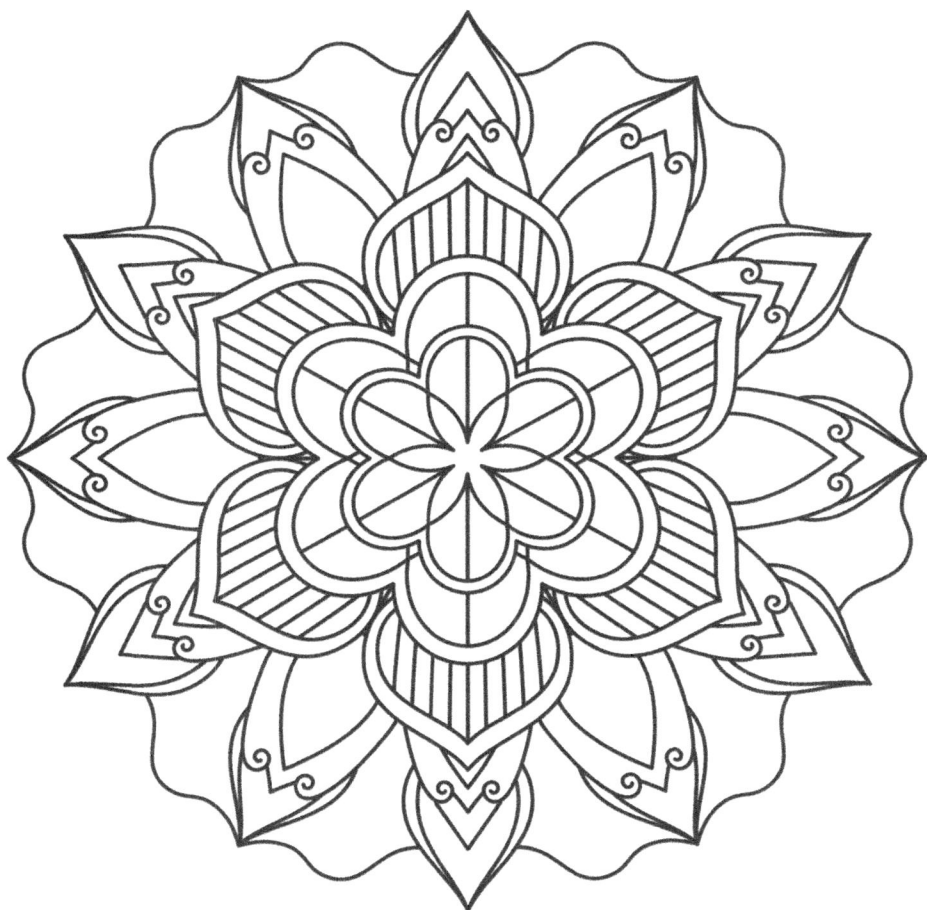

I am always in the right place at the right time

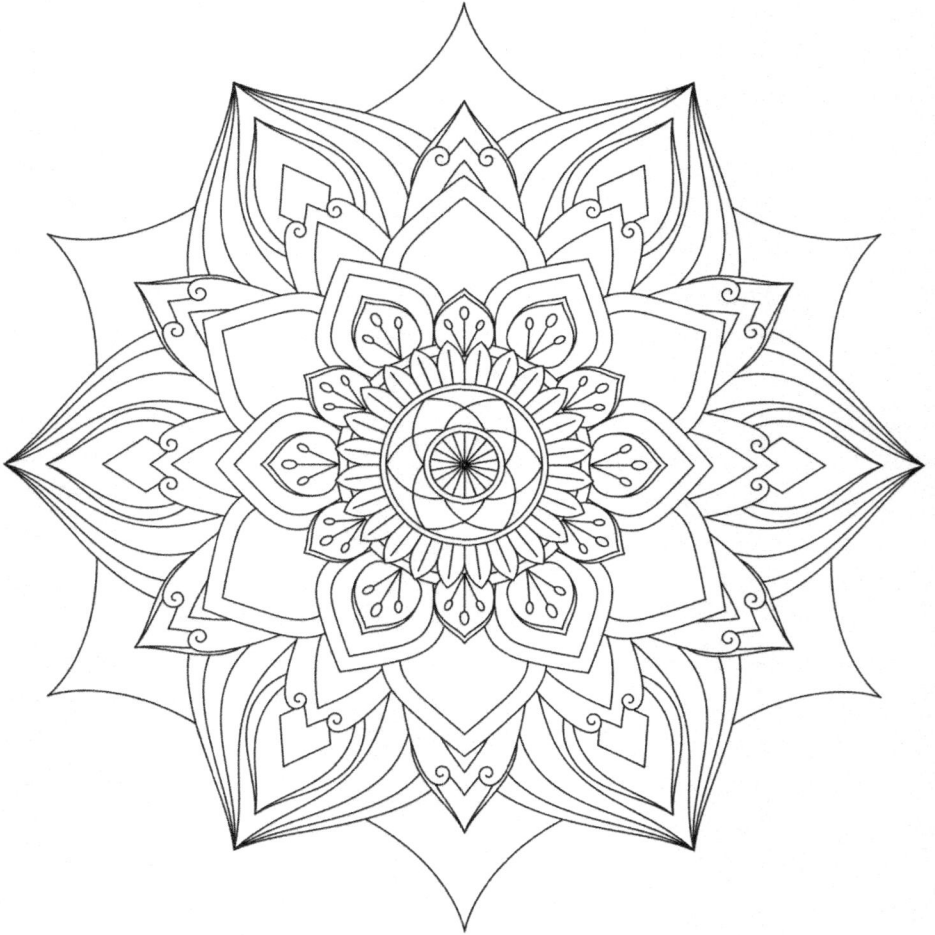

I have everything I need
to overcome this challenge

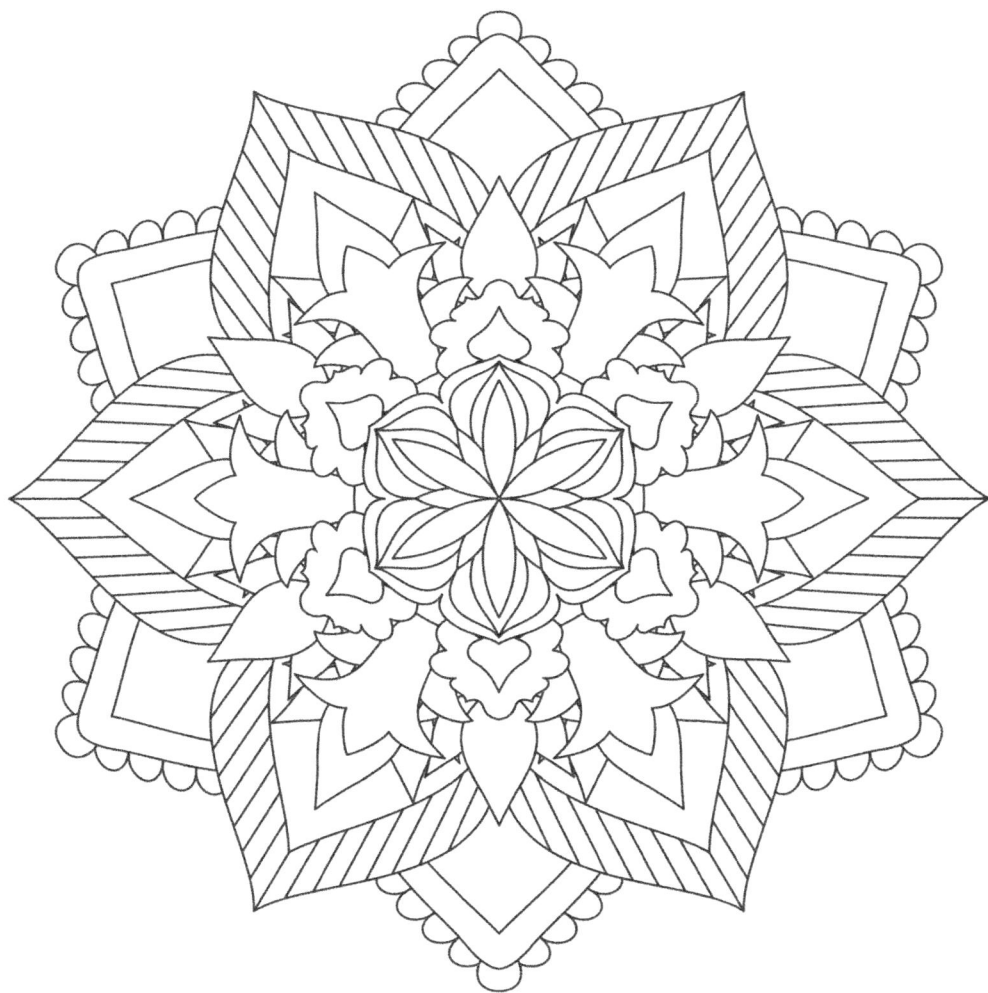

I'm thankful to get to live another day

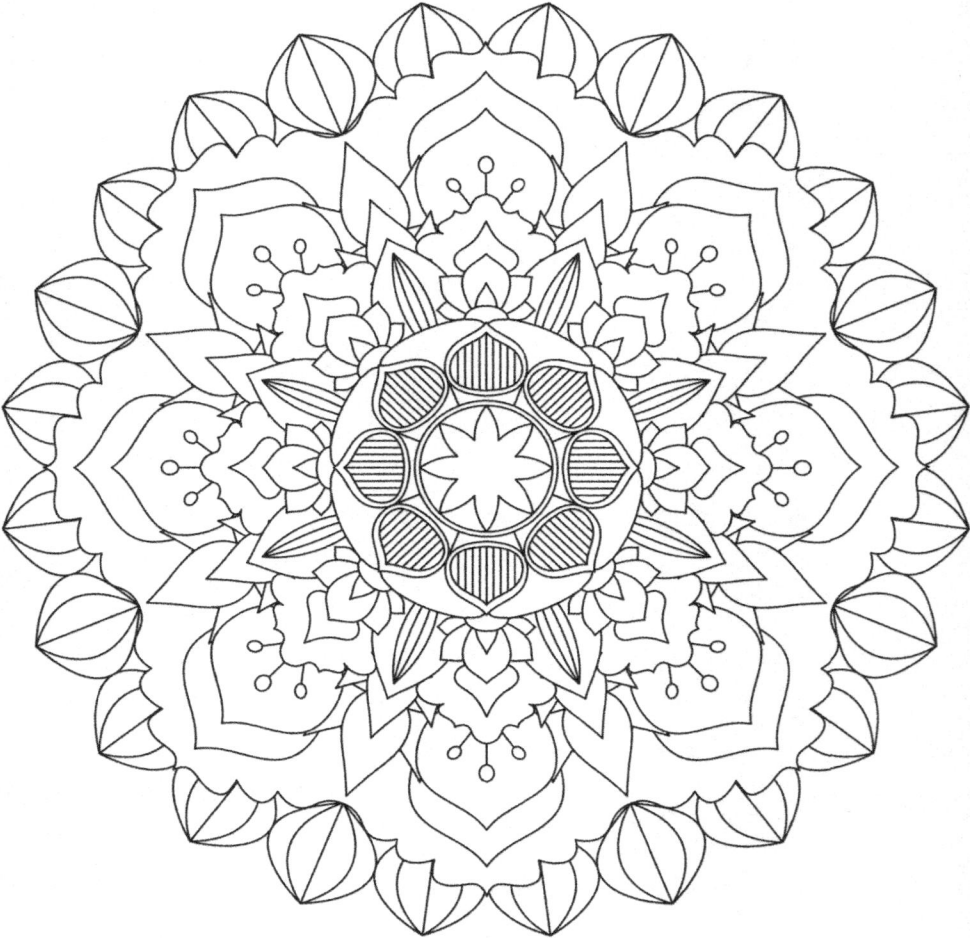

Today I will not stress over things I can't control

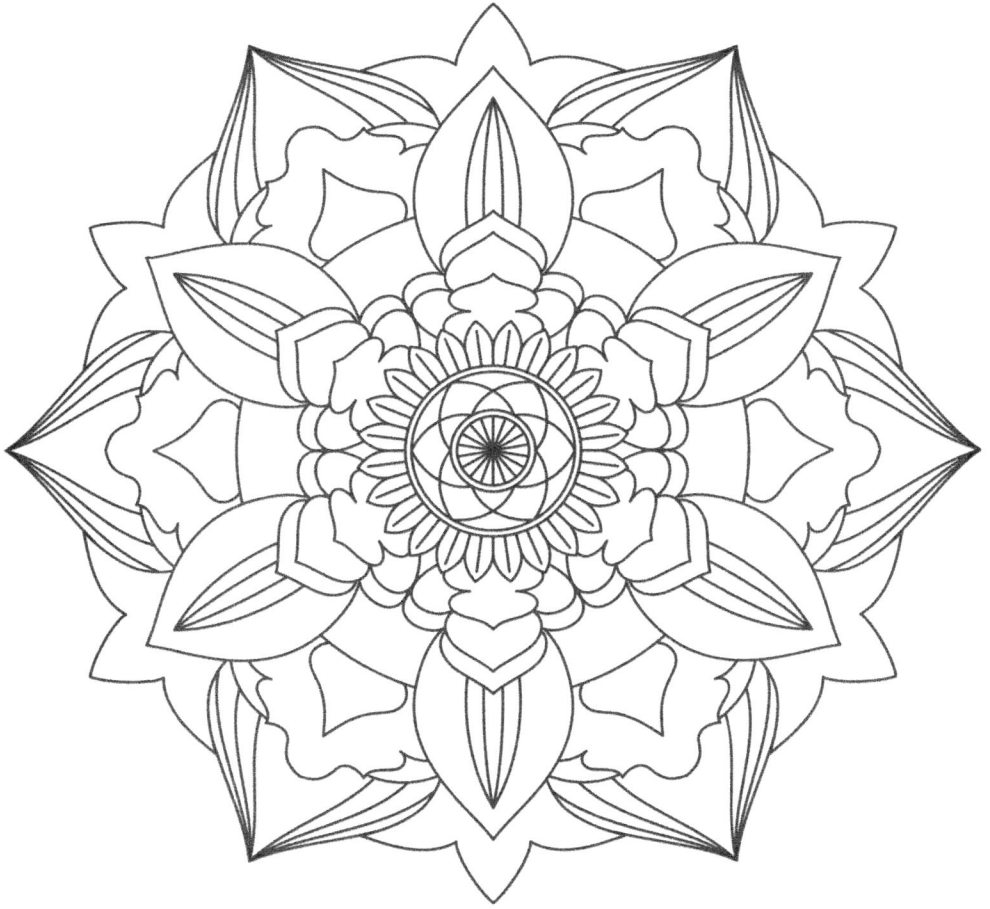

I will focus on what's going right,
Not what's going wrong

_____

_____

_____

_____

_____

_____

_____

_____

_____

_____

_____

_____

_____

_____

_____

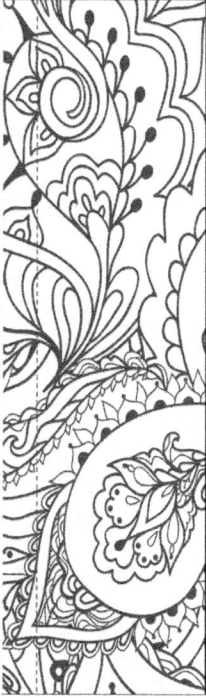

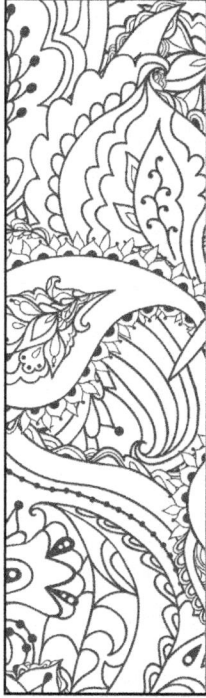

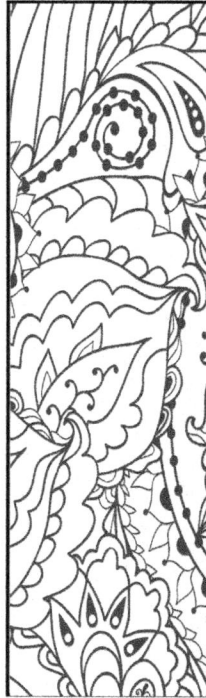

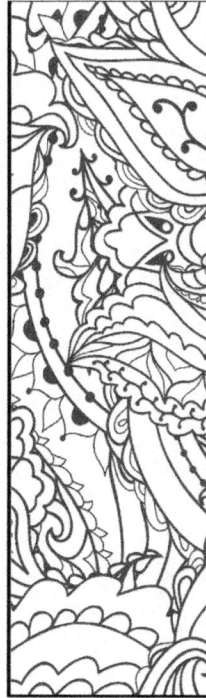

This is only temporary

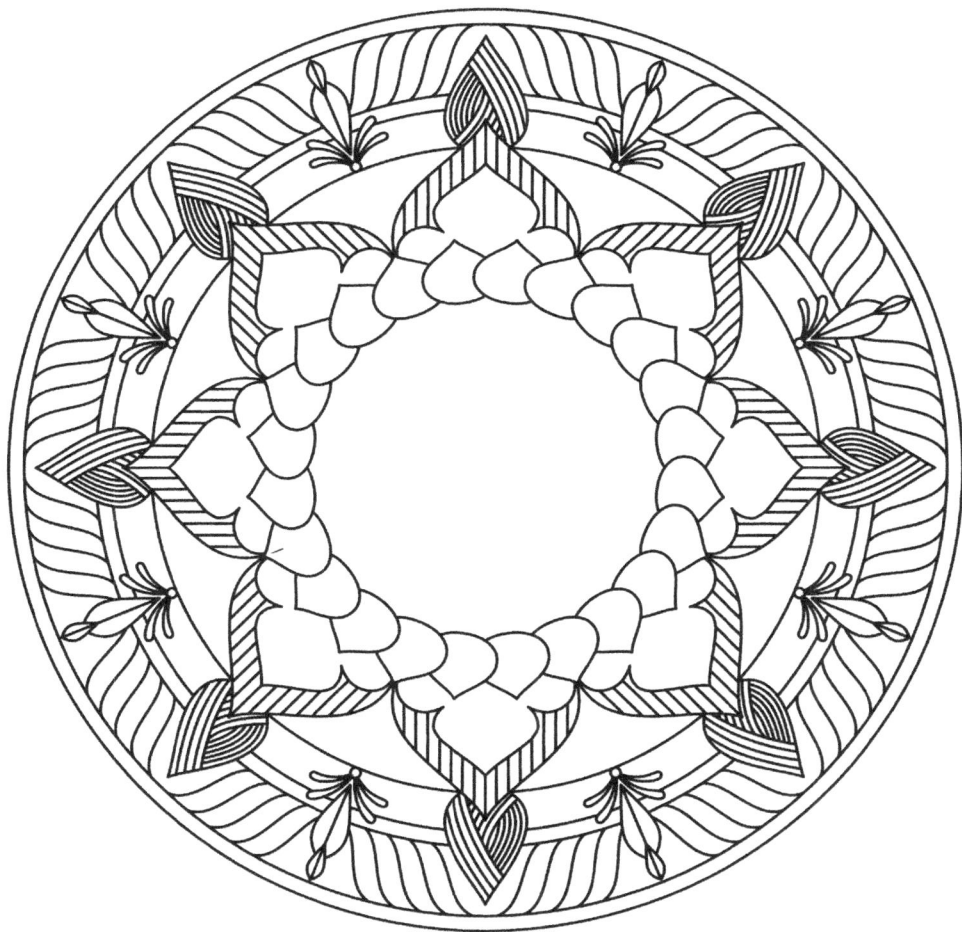

I have the power to change my story

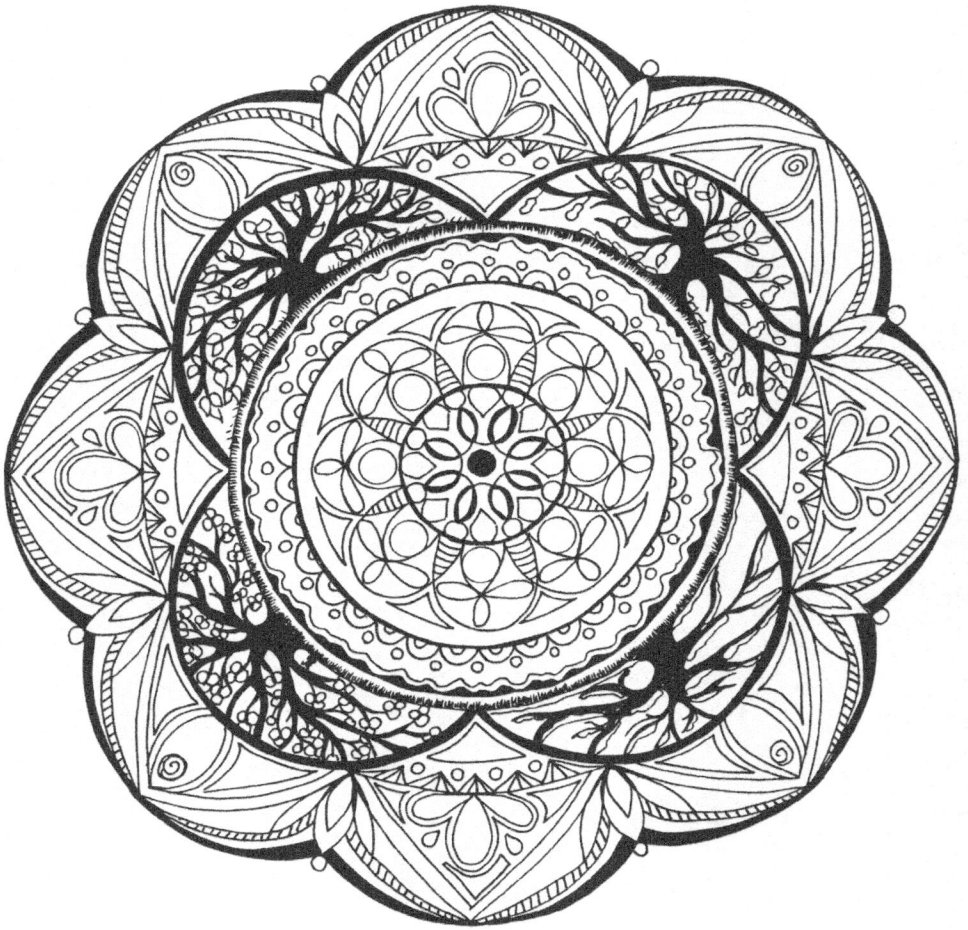

I believe in myself and my abilities

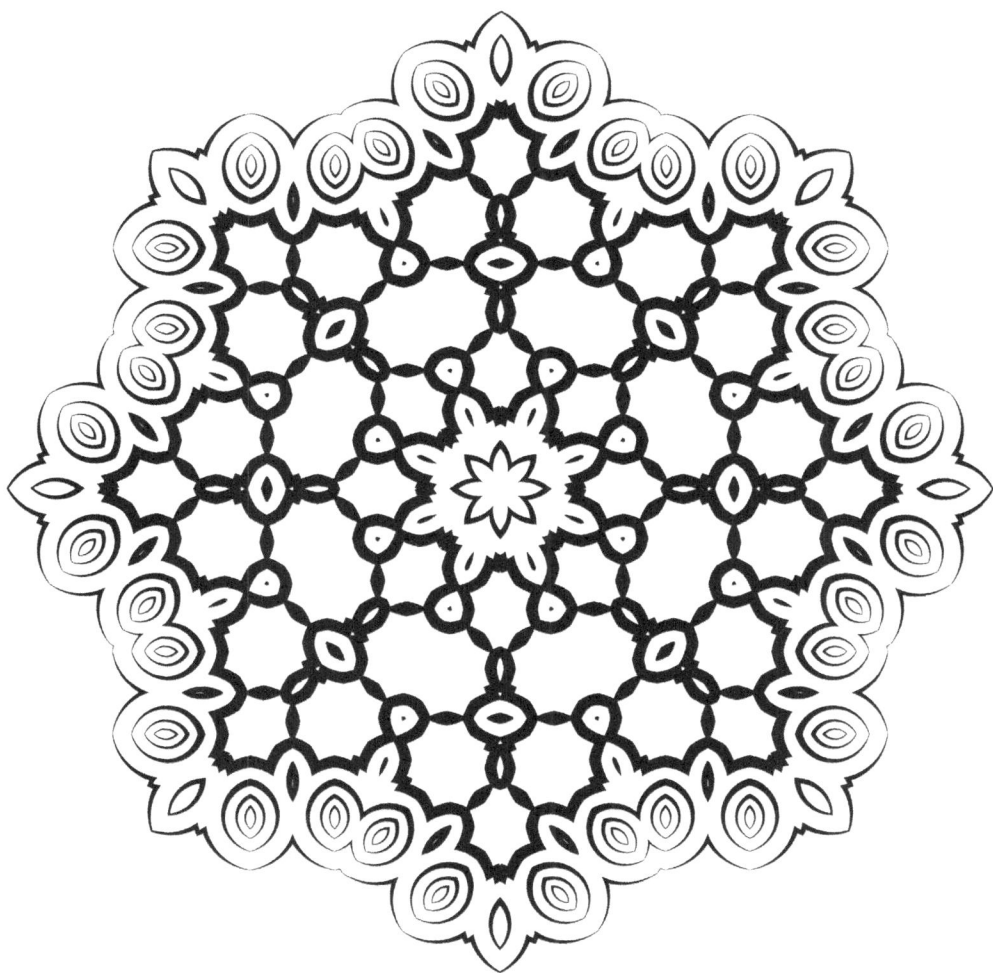

I was not made to give up

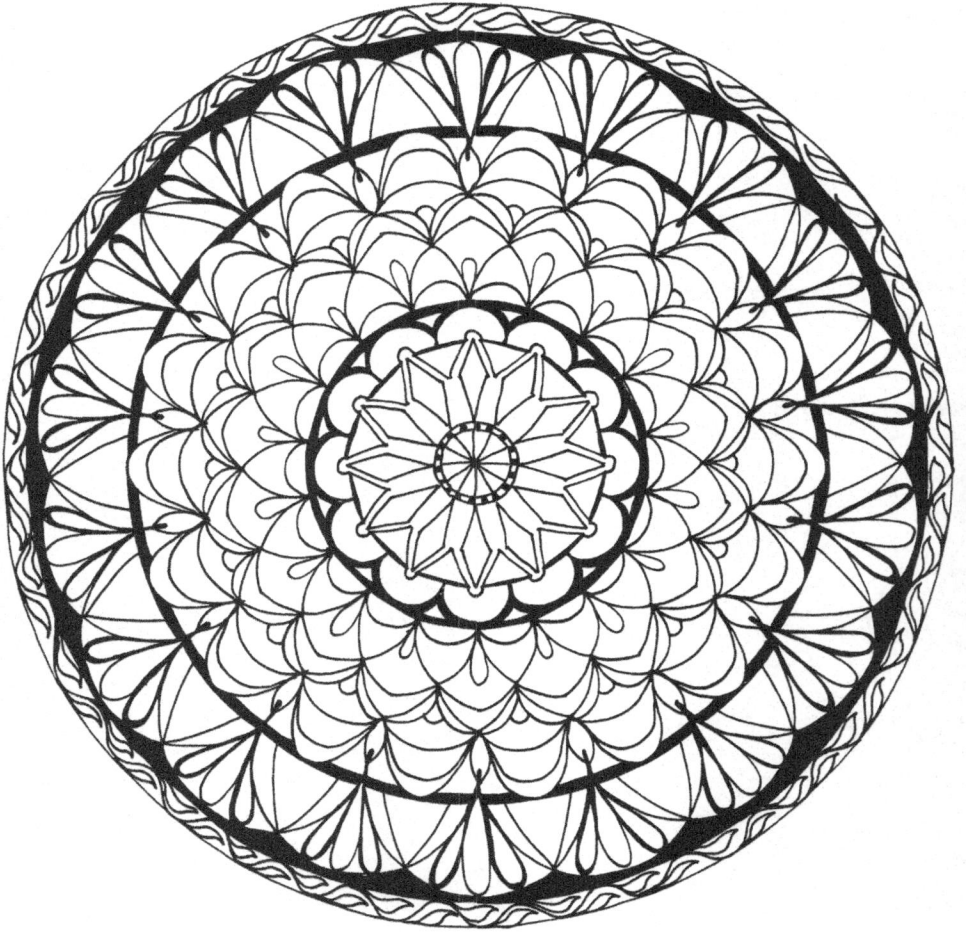

I will bend, so I don't break

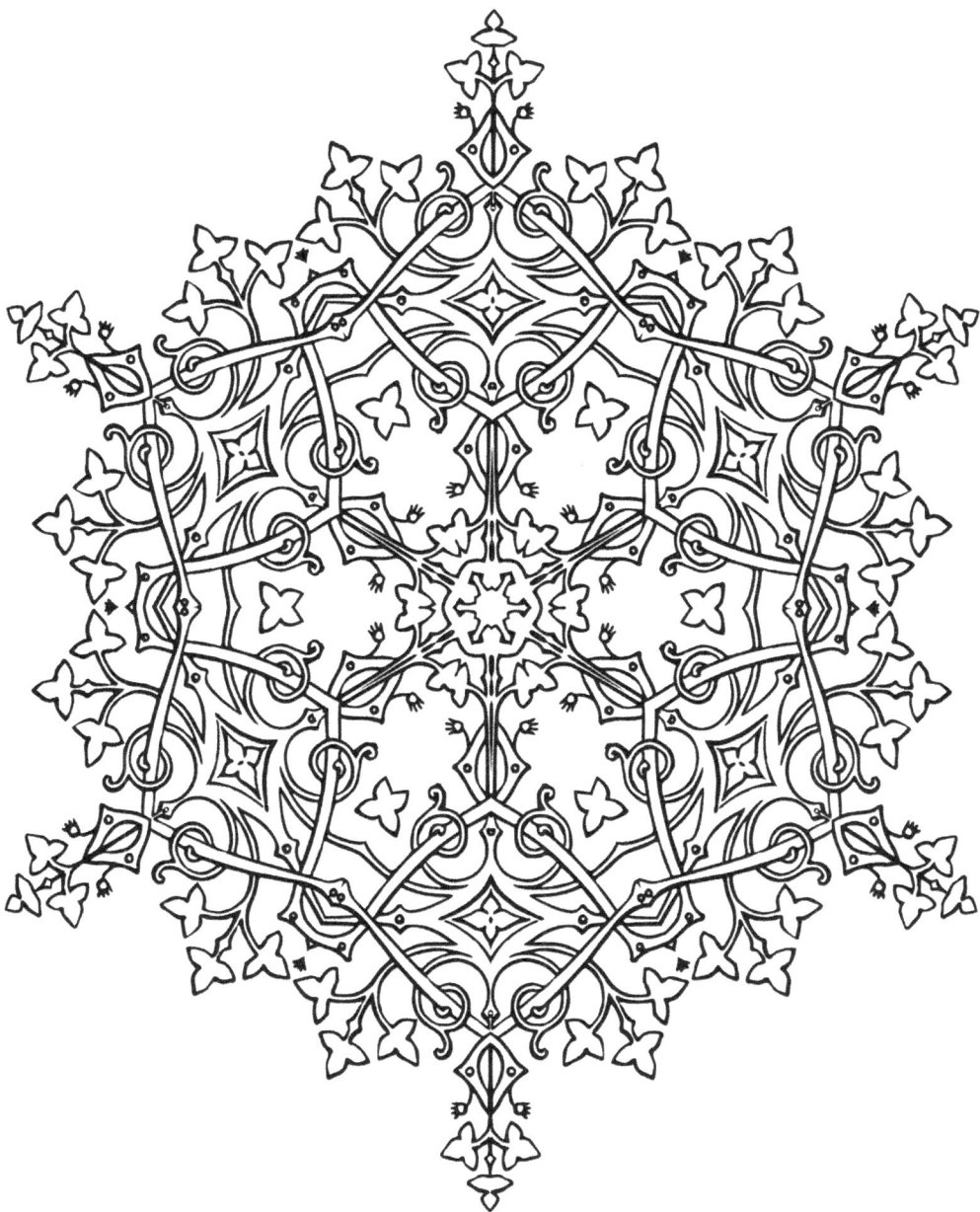

I am fearless and brave

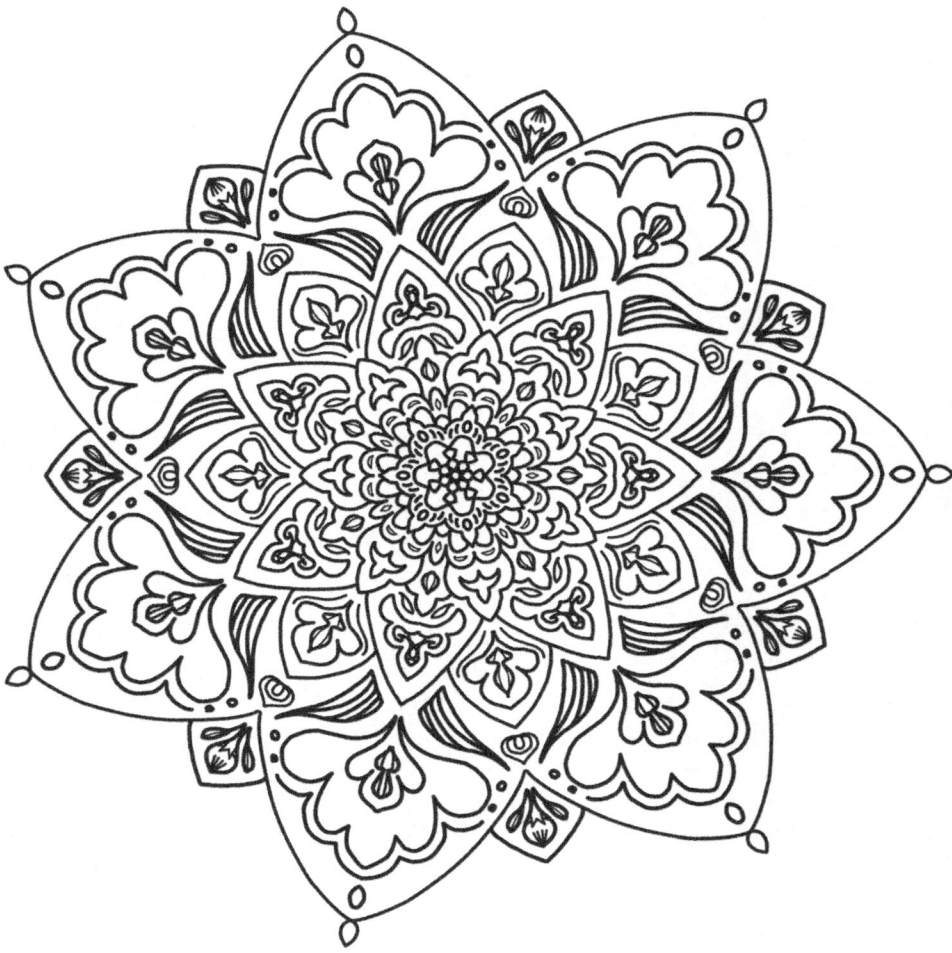

I am proud of myself and my accomplishments

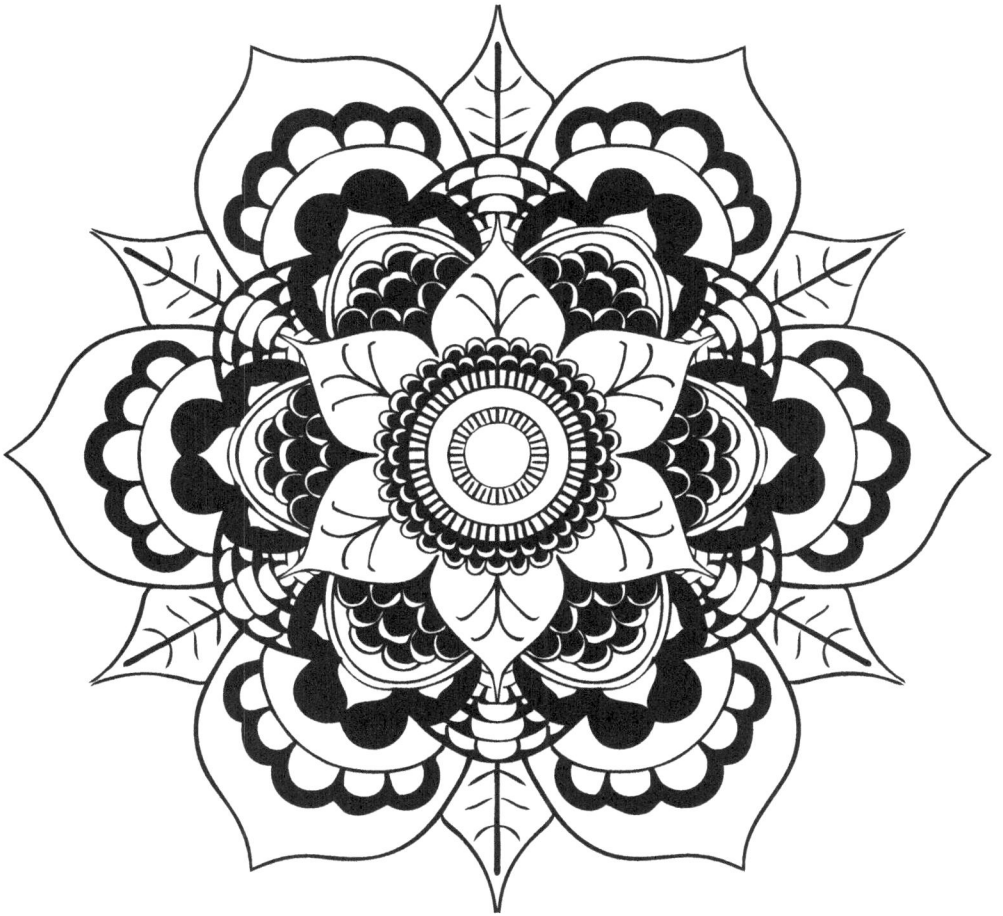

I am in charge of how I feel

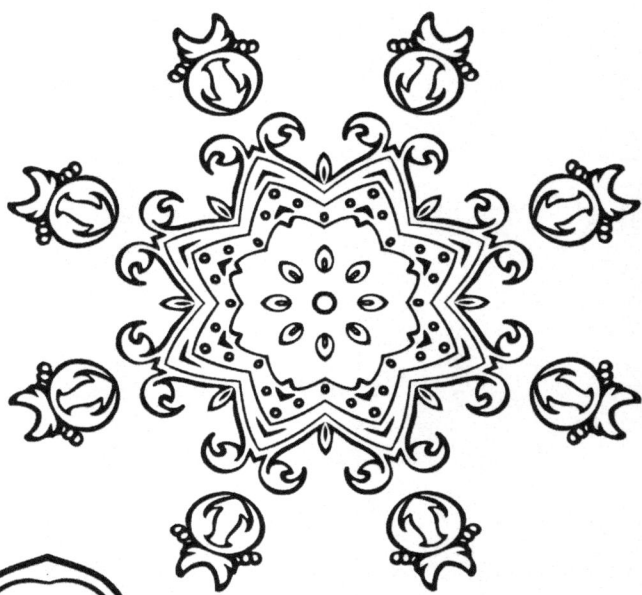

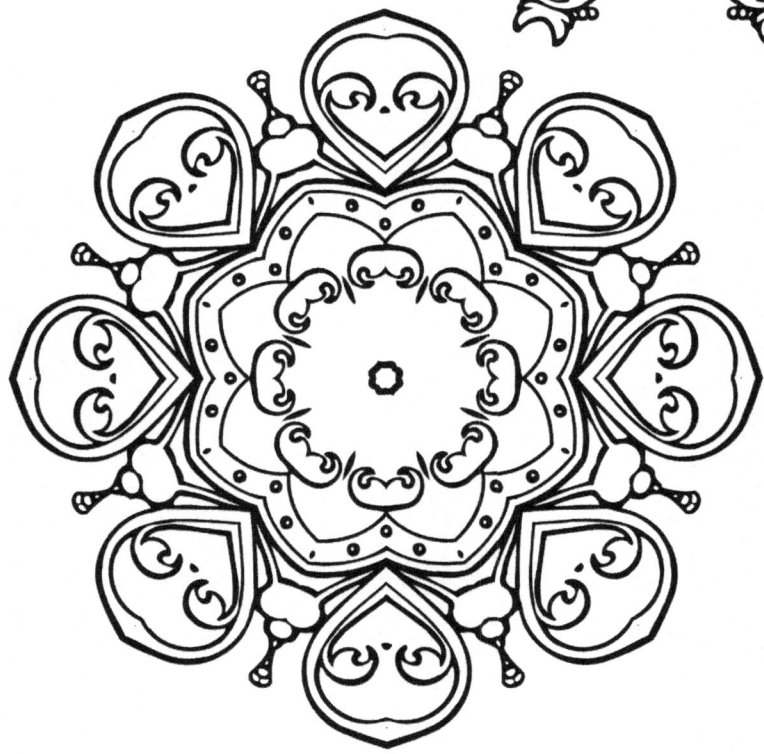

I choose not to take it personally

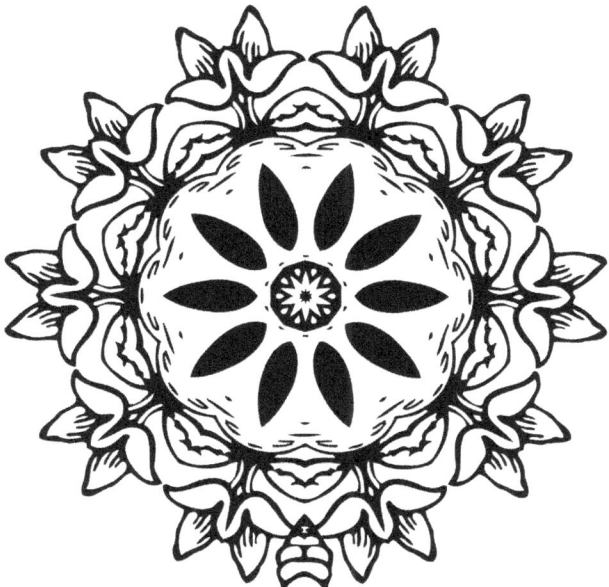

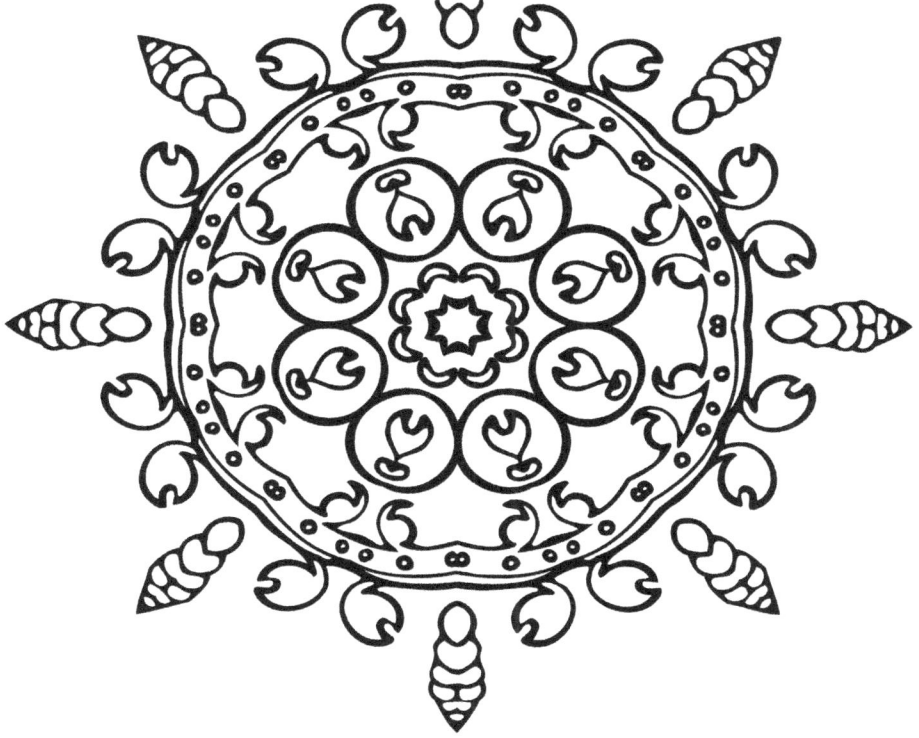

All I need is within me